The Sirtfood Diet Cookbook for Desserts and Snacks

50 quick and healthy recipes to enjoy delicious delicacies

Anne Patel

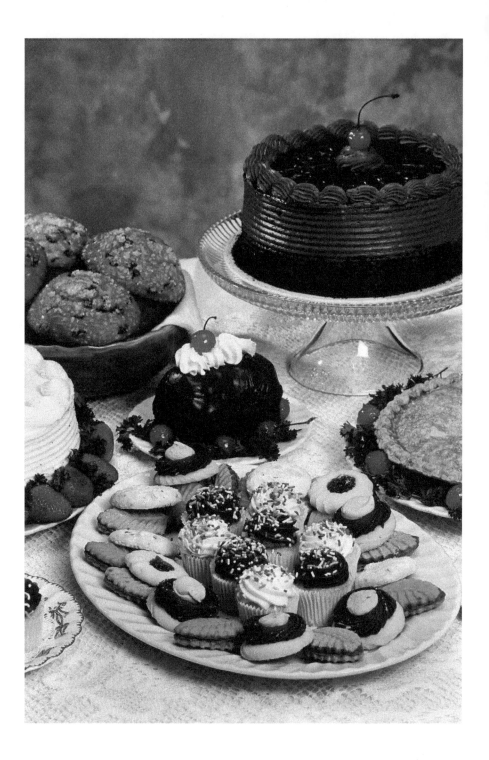

sources. Please consult a licensed professional before attempting any techniques outlined in this book.

By reading this document, the reader agrees that under no circumstances is the author responsible for any losses, direct or indirect, which are incurred as a result of the use of information contained within this document, including, but not limited to, — errors, omissions, or inaccuracies.

Table of Contents

Chapter 1: What is the Sirtfood diet

The Sirtfood Diet was created by Masters in Nutritional Medicine, Aiden Goggins and Glen Matten.

Their goal initially was to find a healthier way for people to eat, but people started losing weight quickly when they tested their program. With all the people in the world following diets hoping to lose pounds, they thought it would be selfish not to disclose their innovative health plan.

The plan they developed focuses on combining certain foods eaten in order to maximize the supply of nutrition to our body. There is an initial phase in which calories are limited to give the body a period to recover and eliminate accumulated waste. A maintenance phase follows this first phase to accustom the metabolism to the new foods you are ingesting. Throughout all stages, you will incorporate potent green juices and well-structured, well-planned meals.

The diet focuses on so-called 'sirtfoods,' plant-based foods that are known to stimulate a gene called sirtuin in the human body.

Sirtuins belong to an entire protein family, called SIRT1 to SIRT7, and each has specific health-related connections. These proteins help separate and safeguard our cells from inflammation and other damage resulting from everyday activities, helping to reduce our risk of developing major diseases, particularly those related to aging.

Studies have shown that people live longer and healthier lives when they eat diets rich in these foods that activate sirtuin, free from diabetes, heart disease, and even dementia. So this diet was designed to restore a healthy body situation, and one of the byproducts of a healthy body is also the loss of excess weight.

The diet Sirtfood is neither a miracle cure nor a week-long program designed to quickly lose weight before beach holidays. If you are only interested in losing a few pounds and then returning to your old habits, there are certainly plans and diets that are more suited to your needs.

The Sirtfood diet is a project born to help you for the rest of your life, using delicious foods, but that will also improve your health. If you switch from a standard American diet (SAD) to a sirtfood diet, you will lose all the weight your body does not need.

A healthy body does not store extra energy. It asks for what it needs and uses it effectively.

The diet isn't designed to encourage you to starve or deprive yourself. The fact is, foods that are deficient in nutrients are designer made to deprive you and, though the calories are there in plenty, your cells are still starved for the nutrition to help you thrive. The Sirtfood Diet is the opposite of deprivation and starvation. It is nourishment and balance.

Most people following the SAD may use 20 ingredients in a month, let alone enjoy the sheer volume of choice ingredients from the 120 options you will learn about here.

In recent decades, an alarming number of people have come to the conclusion that healthy food is boring, and plants or, more specifically, vegetables are terrible tasting. This is because the foods we've become dependent on – packed with sugar, salt, and unhealthy fats – have chemically altered our connection to food. Our brains are essentially lying to us, and our taste buds have been compromised.

This is one of the reasons the week-long reset is so important. After this first week, you will be able to taste food differently. The more you expose yourself to the recommended plant-based foods, the more pleasure you get out of them.

Sirtuins are critical for our health, regulating many essential biological functions, including our metabolism, which, I'm sure you know, is very closely connected to our weight. It's also a key figure in determining our body composition, such as how much muscle we build and how much fat we retain.

Sirtuin genes regulate all this and more. They're also integral in the process of aging and disease.

If we can turn these genes on, we'll be able to protect our cells and enjoy better health for longer life. Eating sirtfoods is the most effective way to accomplish this goal.

Sirtfoods are all plant-based, and they have many more benefits, in addition to being sirtuin activators.

Our bodies require energy to operate, and the majority of this fuel comes from three primary macronutrients: carbohydrates, fats, and proteins. These macros largely control our metabolic system and regulate how the calories we consume get processed by our bodies. This is why most diets focus exclusively on micronutrition and require you to calculate calories.

Our bodies need more than just energy to survive than thriving, however, which is why micronutrients are so important. They don't impact our weight as obviously as macros, but they are our health foundations.

Micronutrients, such as vitamins, minerals, fiber, antioxidants, and phytonutrients, are supposed to be consumed along with our calories. Unfortunately, in the Standard American Diet (SAD), they're in very limited supply.

When your diet is primarily made up of large quantities of red meat and processed meats, pre-packaged foods, vegetable oils, refined grains and a lot of sugar, you will have an almost total lack of micronutrition.

Plant foods offer the most micronutrients per calorie consumed. Every edible plant has a unique nutritional profile, protecting you from an innumerable variety of illnesses.

Sirtfoods, and other plant-based sources of nutrition, give your body what it needs to stay young and disease-free, and, as a bonus, this will help you remain at an ideal weight.

The original Sirtfood Diet encourages you to commit to a one week reset phase and then a 2-week maintenance phase where you rely heavily on the Sirtfood green juice for a significant dose of nutrition along with meals rich in sirtfoods. Once the phases are complete, to retain your health for the rest of your life, you will need to continue incorporating these sirtfoods into your daily meals.

The Sirtfood Diet is not a miracle cure, but if you stick to these recipes, you'll not just impress your taste buds, but you'll also enhance nearly every aspect of your health. To get safe, you don't have to count calories or starve yourself, the youthful body you've always wanted.

Sirtfood Diet Phases

Every newbie needs to understand that the sirtfood diet does not start with a single list of ingredients in your hands. Its implementation and adaptation are more than mere selective grocery shopping. Every diet can only work effectively when we allow our body to embrace the sudden shift and change in food intake. Similarly, the sirtfood diet also comes with two phases of adaptation. If a dieter successfully goes through these phases, he can continue with the sirtfood diet easily. There are mainly two phases of this diet, which are then succeeded by a third phase in which you can decide how you want to continue the diet.

Phase One

The first seven days of this diet plan are characterized as Phase One. In this phase, a dieter must focus on calorie restriction and the intake of green juices. These seven days are crucial to initiate your weight loss and usually help to lose up to seven pounds if the diet is followed properly. If you find yourself achieving this target, that means that you are on the right track.

In the first three days of the first phase, a dieter must restrict this caloric intake to 1,000 calories only. While doing so, the dieter must also have green juice throughout the day, probably three times a day. Try to drink green juice per meal. The recipes given in the book are perfect for selecting from.

Many meal options can keep your caloric intake in checks, such as buckwheat noodles, seared tofu, some shrimp stir fry, or sirtfood omelet.

Once the first three days of this diet has passed, you can increase your caloric intake to 1,500 calories per day. In these next four days, you can reduce the green juices to two times per side. And pair the juices with more Sirtuin-rich food in every meal.

Phase Two

After the first week of the sirtfood diet, then starts phase two. This phase is more about the maintenance of the diet, as the first week enables the body to embrace the change and start working according to the new diet. This phase enables the body to continue working towards the weight loss objective slowly and steadily. Therefore, the duration of this phase is almost two weeks.

So how is this phase different from phase one? In this phase, there is no restriction on the caloric intake, as long as the food is rich in sirtuins and you are taking it three times a day, it is good to go. Instead of having the green juice two or three times a day, the dieter can have juice one time a day, and that will be enough to achieve steady weight loss. You can have the juice after any meal, in the morning or in the evening.

After the Diet Phase

With the end of phase two comes the time, which is most crucial, and that is the after-diet phase. If your weight loss target has not been reached by the end of step two, then you can restart the phases all over again. Or even when you have achieved the goals but still want to lose more weight, then you can again give it a try.

Instead of following phases one and two over and over again, you can also continue having good quality sirtfood meals in this after-diet phase. Simply continue the eating practices of phase two, have a diet rich in sirtuin and do have green juices whenever possible. The diet is mainly divided into two phases: the first lasts one week, and the other lasts 14 days.

The best 20 sirt foods

All these foods include high quantities of plant compounds called polyphenols, which can be thought to modify the sirtuin enzymes, therefore, excite their super-healthy added benefits.

Top 20 sirtfoods

1. Arugula (Rocket)
2. Buckwheat
3. Capers
4. Celery
5. Chilis
6. Cocoa
7. Coffee
8. Extra Virgin Olive Oil
9. Garlic
10. Green Tea (especially Matcha)
11. Kale
12. Medjool Dates
13. Parsley
14. Red Endive
15. Red Onions
16. Red Wine
17. Soy
18. Strawberries

19. Turmeric

20. Walnuts

What Is So Great About Sirtuins?

There are seven types of Sirtuins named from **SIRT1** to **SIRT7**. Although our understanding of the exact functions of all the Sirtuins is minimal, studies show that activating them can have the following benefits:

Switching on fat burning and protection from weight gain: Sirtuins do this by increasing the mitochondrion's functionality (which is involved in the production of energy) and sparking a change in your metabolism to break down more fat cells.

Improving Memory by protecting neurons from damage. Sirtuins also boost learning skills and memory through the enhancement of synaptic plasticity. Synaptic plasticity refers to synapses' capacity to weaken or strengthen with time due to decreased or increased activity. This is important because memories are represented by different interconnected networks of synapses in the brain, and synaptic plasticity is an important neurochemical foundation of memory and learning.

Slowing down the Ageing Process: Sirtuins act as cell guarding enzymes. Thus, they protect the cells and slow down their aging process.

Repairing cells: The Sirtuins repair cells damaged by re-activating cell functionality.

Protection against diabetes: this happens through prevention against insulin resistance. Sirtuins do this by controlling blood sugar levels because this diet calls for moderate consumption of carbohydrates. These foods cause increases in blood sugar levels; hence the need to release insulin, and as the blood sugar levels increase greatly, there is a need to produce more insulin. Over time, cells become resistant to insulin, hence producing more insulin and leading to insulin resistance.

Fighting Cancers: The chemicals working as sirtuin activators affect the function of sirtuin in different cells, i.e. by switching it on when in normal cells and shutting it down in cancerous cells. This encourages the death of cancerous cells.

Fighting inflammation: Sirtuins have a powerful antioxidant effect that has the power to reduce oxidative stress. This has positive effects on heart health and cardiovascular protection.

Chapter 2: How do the Sirtfood Diet Works?

The basis of the sirtuin diet can be explained in simple terms or in complex ways. However, it's important to understand how and why it works so that you can appreciate the value of what you are doing. It is important to also know why these sirtuin rich foods help to help you maintain fidelity to your diet plan. Otherwise, you may throw something in your meal with less nutrition that would defeat the purpose of planning for one rich in sirtuins. Most importantly, this is not a dietary fad, and as you will see, there is much wisdom contained in how humans have used natural foods, even for medicinal purposes, over thousands of years.

To understand how the Sirtfood diet works and why these particular foods are necessary, we're going to look at their role in the human body.

Sirtuin activity was first researched in yeast, where a mutation caused an extension in the yeast's lifespan. Sirtuins were also shown to slow aging in laboratory mice, fruit flies, and nematodes. As research on Sirtuins proved to transfer to mammals, they were examined for their use in diet and slowing the aging process. The sirtuins in humans are different in typing, but they essentially work in the same ways and reasons.

The Sirtuin family is made up of seven "members." It is believed that sirtuins play a big role in regulating certain functions of cells, including proliferation, reproduction and growth of cells), apoptosis death of cells). They promote survival and resist stress to increase longevity.

They are also seen to block neurodegeneration loss or function of the nerve cells in the brain). They conduct their housekeeping functions by cleaning out toxic proteins and supporting the brain's ability to change and adapt to different conditions or to recuperate i.e., brain plasticity). They also help minimize chronic inflammation as part of this and decrease anything called oxidative stress. Oxidative stress is when there are so many free radicals present in the body that are cell-damaging, and by fighting them with antioxidants, the body can not keep up. These factors are related to age-related illness and weight as well, which again brings us back to a discussion of how they actually work.

You will see labels in Sirtuins that start with "SIR," which represents "Silence Information Regulator" genes. They do exactly that, silence or regulate, as part of their functions. Humans work with the seven sirtuins: SIRT1, SIRT2, SIRT3,

SIRT4, SIRT 5, SIRT6 and SIRT7. Each of these types is responsible for different areas of protecting cells. They work by either stimulating or turning on certain gene expressions or by reducing and turning off other gene expressions. This essentially means that they can influence genes to do more or less of something, most of which they are already programmed to do.

Through enzyme reactions, each of the SIRT types affects different areas of cells responsible for the metabolic processes that help maintain life. This is also related to what organs and functions they will affect.

For example, the SIRT6 causes and expression of genes in humans that affect skeletal muscle, fat tissue, brain, and heart. SIRT 3 would cause an expression of genes that affect the kidneys, liver, brain and heart.

If we tie these concepts together, you can see that the Sirtuin proteins can change the expression of genes, and in the case of the Sirtfood diet, we care about how sirtuins can turn off those genes that are responsible for speeding up aging and for weight management.

The other aspect to this conversation of sirtuins is the function and the power of calorie restriction on the human body. Calorie restriction is simply eating fewer calories. This, coupled with exercise and reducing stress, is usually a combination for weight loss. Calorie restriction has also proven across much research in animals and humans to increase one's lifespan.

We can look further at the role of sirtuins with calorie restriction and using the SIRT3 protein, which has a role in metabolism and aging. Amongst all of the effects of the protein on gene expression, such as preventing cells from dying, reducing tumors from growing, etc.), we want to understand the effects of SIRT3 on weight for this book's purpose.

As we stated earlier, the SIRT3 has high expression in those metabolically active tissues, and its ability to express itself increases with caloric restriction, fasting, and exercise. On the contrary, it will express itself less when the body has high fat, high calorie-riddled diet.

The last few highlights of sirtuins are their role in regulating telomeres and reducing inflammation, which also helps with staving off disease and aging.
Telomeres are sequences of proteins at the ends of chromosomes. When cells divide, these get shorter. As we age, they get shorter, and other stressors to the body also will contribute to this. Maintaining these longer telomeres is the key to slower aging. In addition, proper diet, along with exercise and other variables, can lengthen telomeres. SIRT6 is one of the

sirtuins that, if activated, can help with DNA damage, inflammation and oxidative stress. SIRT1 also helps with inflammatory response cycles that are related to many age-related diseases.

Calories restriction can extend life to some degree. Since this and fasting are a stressor, these factors will stimulate the SIRT3 proteins to kick in and protect the body from the stressors and excess free radicals. Again, the telomere length is affected as well.

Having laid this all out before you, you should appreciate how and why these miraculous compounds work in your favor, keep you youthful, healthy, and lean If they are working hard for you, don't you feel that you should do something too?

50 Desserts and Snacks Recipes

1. Chocolate Granola

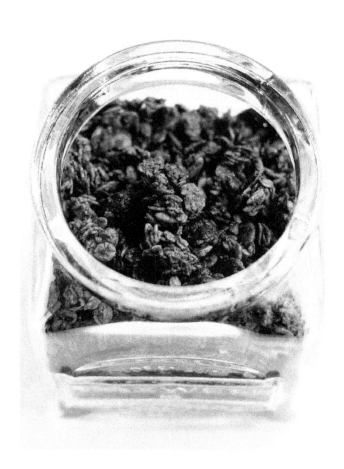

Preparation time: 10 minutes

Cooking time: 38 minutes

Total time: 48 minutes

Servings: 8

Ingredients:

¼ cup cacao powder

¼ cup maple syrup

2 tablespoons coconut oil, melted

½ teaspoon vanilla extract

1/8 teaspoon salt

2 cups gluten-free rolled oats

¼ cup unsweetened coconut flakes

2 tablespoons chia seeds

2 tablespoons unsweetened dark chocolate, chopped finely

Directions:

1. Preheat your oven to 300oF and use parchment paper to line a medium baking sheet.

2. In a medium pan, add the cacao powder, maple syrup, coconut oil, vanilla extract, and salt, and mix well.

3. Now, over medium heat, position the pan and cook for about 2-3 minutes, or, stirring continuously, until thick and syrupy.

4. Remove from the heat and set aside.

5. Then add the oats, coconut, and chia seeds to a wide bowl and combine well.

6. Add the syrup mixture and mix until well combined.

7. Transfer the granola mixture onto a prepared baking sheet and spread in an even layer.

8. Bake for about 35 minutes.

9. Remove from the oven and leave for around 1 hour to set aside.

10. Add the chocolate pieces and stir to combine.
11. Serve immediately.

Nutrition:
Calories 193
Sodium: 24 mg
Dietary Fiber: 1.7 g
Total Fat: 3.1 g

Total Carbs: 16.7 g

Protein: 1.5 g

2. Homemade Marshmallow Fluff

Preparation time: 10 minutes

Cooking time: 20 minutes

Servings: 2

Ingredients:

3/4 cup sugar

1/2 cup light corn syrup

1/4 cup water

⅛ teaspoon salt

3 little egg whites

1/4 teaspoon cream of tartar

1 teaspoon 1/2 tsp vanilla extract

Directions:

1. In a little pan, mix together sugar, corn syrup, salt and water. Attach a candy thermometer into the side of this pan, but make sure it will not touch the underside of the pan.

2. From the bowl of a stand mixer, combine egg whites and cream of tartar. Begin to whip on medium speed with the whisk attachment.

3. Meanwhile, turn a burner on top and place the pan with the sugar mix onto heat. Put the mix into a boil and heat to 240 degrees, stirring periodically.

4. The aim is to have the egg whites whipped to soft peaks and also the sugar heated to 240 degrees at near the same moment. Simply stop stirring the egg whites once they hit soft peaks.

5. Once the sugar has already reached 240 amounts, turn heat low, allowing it to reduce. Insert a little quantity of the popular sugar mix and let it mix. Insert still another little sum of the sugar mix. Add mix slowly and that means you never scramble the egg whites.

6. After all of the sugar was added into the egg whites, then decrease the speed of the mixer and also keep mixing concoction for around 7- 9 minutes until the fluff remains glossy and stiff. At roughly the 5-minute mark, then add the vanilla extract.

7. Use fluff immediately or store in an airtight container in the fridge for around two weeks.

Nutrition:
Calories: 159
Sodium: 32 mg
Dietary Fiber: 1.5 g

Total Fat: 3.1 g

Total Carbs: 15.3 g

Protein: 1.4 g

3. Ultimate Chocolate Chip Cookie N' Oreo Fudge Brownie Bar

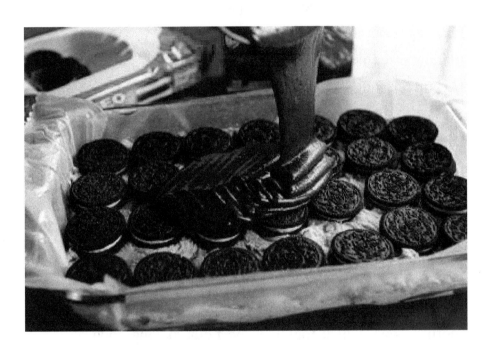

Preparation time: 10 minutes

Cooking time: 50 minutes

Servings: 2

Ingredients:

1 cup (2 sticks) butter, softened

1 cup granulated sugar

3/4 cup light brown sugar

2 large egg

1 tablespoon pure vanilla extract

2 ½ cups all-purpose flour

1 teaspoon baking soda

1 teaspoon lemon

2 cups (12 oz) milk chocolate chips

1 package double stuffed Oreo

1 family-size (9×1 3) brownie mixture

1/4 cup hot fudge topping

Directions:

1. Preheat oven to 350 degrees F.

2. Cream the butter and sugar in a wide bowl and use a medium-speed electric mixer for 35 minutes.

3. To blend completely, add the vanilla and eggs and mix well. In another bowl, whisk together the flour, baking soda and salt, and slowly incorporate in the mixer everything is combined.

4. Stir in chocolate chips.

5. Spread the cookie dough at the bottom of a 9×1-3 baking dish that is wrapped with wax paper and then coated with cooking spray.

6. Shirt with a coating of Oreos. Mix together brownie mix, adding an optional 1/4 cup of hot fudge directly into the mixture.

7. Stir the brownie batter within the cookie-dough and Oreos.

8. Cover with foil and bake at 350 degrees F for 30 minutes.

9. Remove foil and continue baking for another 15 25 minutes.

10. Let cool before cutting on brownies. They may be gooey at the while warm but will also set up perfectly once chilled.

Nutrition:
Calories: 145,
Sodium: 33 mg,
Dietary Fiber: 1.4 g,
Total Fat: 4.1 g,
Total Carbs: 16.7 g,
Protein: 1.3 g.

4. Crunchy Chocolate Chip Coconut Macadamia Nut Cookies

Preparation time: 20 minutes

Cooking time: 0 minute

Servings: 2

Ingredients:

1 cup yogurt

1 cup yogurt

1/2 teaspoon baking soda

1/2 teaspoon salt

1 tablespoon of butter, softened

1 cup firmly packed brown sugar

1/2 cup sugar

1 large egg

1/2 cup semi-sweet chocolate chips

1/2 cup sweetened flaked coconut

1/2 cup coarsely chopped dry-roasted macadamia nuts 1/2 cup raisins

Directions:

1. Preheat the oven to 325°f.

2. Whisk together the rice, oatmeal, baking soda and salt in a small cup, then set aside.

3. In your mixer bowl, mix together the butter/sugar/egg mix.

4. Mix in the flour/oats mix until just combined and stir in the chocolate chips, raisins, nuts, and coconut.

5. Place outsized bits on a parchment-lined cookie sheet.

6. Bake for 1-3 minutes before biscuits are only barely golden brown.

7. Remove from the oven and then leave the cookie sheets to cool at least 10 minutes.

Nutrition:
Calories: 167
Sodium: 31 mg
Dietary Fiber: 1.4 g
Total Fat: 4.1 g
Total Carbs: 16.5 g
Protein: 1.3 g

5. Walnut & Date Loaf

Preparation Time: 10 minutes

Cooking Time: 15 minutes

Servings: 12

Ingredients:

9 ounces of self-rising flour

4 ounces of Medrol dates, chopped

2 ounces of walnuts, chopped

8fl oz. milk

3 eggs

1 medium banana, mashed

1 teaspoon baking soda

Directions:

1. In a cup, sieve the baking soda and flour.

2. Add in the banana, eggs, milk and dates and combine all the ingredients thoroughly.

3. Move and smooth out the mixture to a lined loaf tin.

4. Scatter the walnuts on top.

5. Bake the loaf in the oven at 180C/360F for 45 minutes.

6. Serve!

Nutrition:

Calories: 204

Sodium: 33 mg

Dietary Fiber: 1.7 g

Total Fat: 3.1 g

Total Carbs: 16.5 g

Protein: 1.4 g

6. Peach and Blueberry Pie

Preparation time: 1 hour

Cooking time: 0 minute

Servings: 2

Ingredients:

1 box of noodle dough

Filling:

5 peaches, peeled and chopped (I used roasted peaches)

3 cups strawberries

3/4 cup sugar

1/4 cup bread

Juice of 1/2 lemon

1 egg yolk, beaten

Directions:

1. Preheat oven to 400 degrees.

2. Place dough to a 9-inch pie plate

3. In a big bowl, combine tomatoes, sugar, bread, and lemon juice, then toss to combine. Pour into the pie plate, mounding at the center.

4. Simply take some of the bread and then cut into bits, then put a pie shirt and put the dough in addition to pressing on the edges.

5. Brush crust with egg wash then sprinkles with sugar.

6. Set onto a parchment paper-lined baking sheet.

7. Cook for about 20 minutes at 400 o'clock, until the crust is browned at the border.

8. Turn oven down to 350, bake for another 40 minutes.

9. Remove and let sit at least 30minutes.

10. Have with vanilla ice-cream.

Nutrition:
Calories: 167
Sodium: 31 mg
Dietary Fiber: 1.4 g
Total Fat: 4.1 g
Total Carbs: 16.6 g
Protein: 1.2 g

7. Pear, Cranberry and Chocolate Crisp

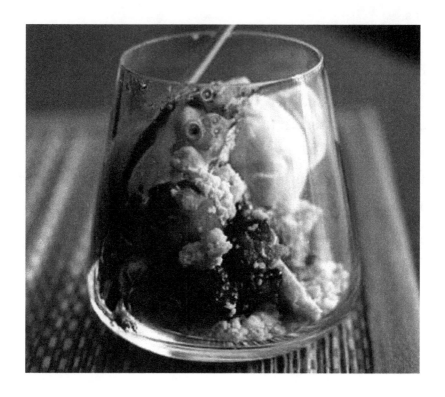

Preparation time: 10 minutes

Cooking time: 20 minutes

Servings: 3

Ingredients:

Crumble topping:

1/2 cup flour

1/2 cup brown sugar

1 tsp cinnamon

⅛ teaspoon salt

3/4 cup yogurt

1/4 cup sliced peppers

1/3 cup butter, melted

1 teaspoon vanilla

Filling:

1 tablespoon brown sugar

3 teaspoons, cut into balls

1/4 cup dried cranberries

1 teaspoon lemon juice

Two handfuls of milk chocolate chips

Directions:

1. Preheat oven to 375.

2. Using butter spray to spray a casserole dish.

3. Put all of the topping ingredients - flour, sugar, cinnamon, salt, nuts, legumes and dried

4. Butter a bowl and then mix. Set aside.

5. Combine the sugar, lemon juice, pears, and cranberries in a wide dish.

6. Once the fully blended move to the prepared baking dish.

7. Spread the topping evenly over the fruit.

8. Bake for about half an hour.

9. Disperse chocolate chips out at the top.

10. Cook for another 10 minutes.

11. Have with ice cream.

Nutrition:

Calories: 324

Sodium: 33 mg

Dietary Fiber: 1.4 g

Total Fat: 4.1 g

Total Carbs: 15.3 g

Protein: 1.3 g

8. Apricot Oatmeal Cookies

Preparation time: 10 minutes

Cooking time: 20 minutes

Servings: 3

Ingredients:

1/2 cup (1 stick) butter, softened

2/3 cup light brown sugar packed

1 egg

3/4 cup all-purpose flour

1/2 teaspoon baking soda

1/2 teaspoon vanilla extract

1/2 teaspoon cinnamon

1/4 teaspoon salt

1 teaspoon 1/2 cups chopped oats

3/4 cup yolks

1/4 cup sliced apricots

1/3 cup slivered almonds

Directions:

1. Preheat oven to 350°.

2. In a big bowl, combine with the butter, sugar, and egg until smooth.

3. In another bowl, whisk the flour, baking soda, cinnamon, and salt together.

4. Stir the dry ingredients to the butter-sugar bowl.

5. Now stir in the oats, raisins, apricots, and almonds.

6. I heard on the web that in this time, it's much better to cool with the dough (therefore, your biscuits are thicker)

7. Afterward, I scooped my biscuits into some parchment-lined (easier removal and wash up) cookie sheet - around two inches apart.

8. Sliced mine for approximately ten minutes - they were fantastic!

Nutrition:

Calories: 132

Sodium: 33 mg

Dietary Fiber: 1.4 g

Total Fat: 3.1 g

Total Carbs: 16.4 g

Protein: 1.3 g

9. Blueberry Muffins

Preparation time: 15 minutes

Cooking time: 20 minutes

Total time: 35 minutes

Servings: 8

Ingredients:

1 cup buckwheat flour

¼ cup arrowroot starch

1½ teaspoons baking powder

¼ teaspoon sea salt

2 eggs

½ cup unsweetened almond milk

2–3 tablespoons maple syrup

2 tablespoons coconut oil, melted

1 cup fresh blueberries

Directions:

1. Preheat your oven to 3500F and put a muffin tin into 8 cups.

2. In a bowl, place the buckwheat flour, arrowroot starch, baking powder, and salt, and mix well.

3. In a separate bowl, place the eggs, almond milk, maple syrup, and coconut oil, and beat until well combined.

4. Now, place the flour mixture and mix until just combined.

5. Gently, fold in the blueberries.

6. Transfer the mixture into prepared muffin cups evenly.

7. Bake for about 25 minutes or until a toothpick inserted in the center comes out clean.

8. Remove the muffin tin from the oven and position it for about 10 minutes on a wire rack to cool.

9. Carefully invert the muffins onto the wire rack to cool completely before serving.

Nutrition:
Calories 136
Sodium: 33 mg
Dietary Fiber: 2.4 g
Total Fat: 4.5 g
Total Carbs: 16.4 g
Protein: 1.2 g

10. Chocolate Waffles

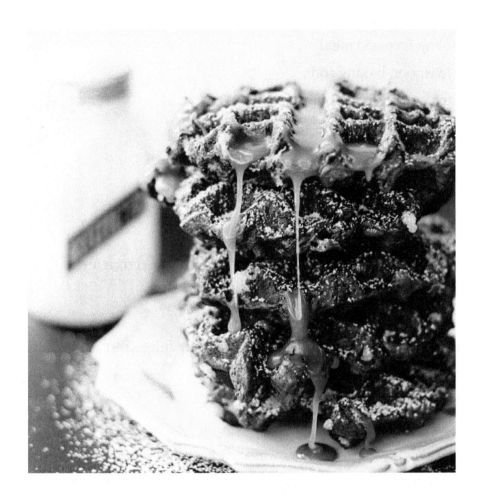

Preparation time: 15 minutes

Cooking time: 24 minutes

Total time: 39 minutes

Servings: 8

Ingredients:

2 cups unsweetened almond milk

1 tablespoon fresh lemon juice

1 cup buckwheat flour

½ cup cacao powder

¼ cup flaxseed meal

1 teaspoon baking soda

1 teaspoon baking powder

¼ teaspoons kosher salt

2 large eggs

½ cup coconut oil, melted

¼ cup dark brown sugar

2 teaspoons vanilla extract

2 ounces unsweetened dark chocolate, chopped roughly

Directions:

1. Put the almond milk and the lemon juice into a bowl and combine well.

2. Set aside for about 10 minutes.

3. In a bowl, place buckwheat flour, cacao powder, flaxseed meal, baking soda, baking powder, and salt, and mix well.

4. In the bowl of the almond milk mixture, place the eggs, coconut oil, brown sugar, and vanilla extract, and beat until smooth.

5. Now, place the flour mixture and beat until smooth.

6. Gently fold in the chocolate pieces.

7. Preheat and then grease the waffle iron.

8. Place the desired amount of the mixture into the preheated waffle iron and cook for about 3 minutes, or until golden-brown.

9. Repeat with the remaining mixture.

Nutrition:
Calories 295
Sodium: 28 mg
Dietary Fiber: 1.8 g
Total Fat: 3.3 g
Total Carbs: 14.2 g
Protein: 1.4 g

11. Snowflakes

Preparation time: 10 minutes
Cooking time: 0 minute
Servings: 2

Ingredients:
Won ton wrappers
Oil for frying
Powdered sugar

Directions:
1. Cut won ton wrappers just like you'd a snowflake

2. Heat oil. When hot, add wonton, fry for approximately 30 seconds, then flips over.

3. Drain it with powdered sugar on a paper towel and dust.

Nutrition:
Calories: 104
Sodium: 37 mg
Dietary Fiber: 1.3 g
Total Fat: 4.6 g
Total Carbs: 15.6 g

Protein: 1.5 g

12. Guilt Totally Free Banana Ice-Cream

Preparation time: 20 minutes

Cooking time: 0 minute

Serves: 3

Ingredients:

3 quite ripe banana - peeled and chopped A couple of chocolate chips

2 tablespoons skim milk

Directions:

1. In a food processor, throw all ingredients and blend until smooth.

2. Eat: freeze and appreciate afterward.

Nutrition:

Calories: 208

Sodium: 33 mg

Dietary Fiber: 1.6 g

Total Fat: 2.6 g

Total Carbs: 14.6 g

Protein: 1.8 g

13. Mascarpone Cheesecake With Almond Crust

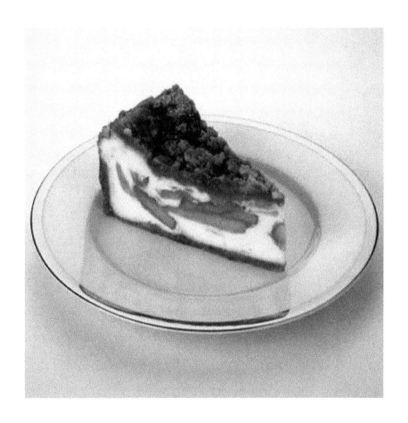

Preparation time: 10 minutes

Cooking time: 0 minute

Servings: 2

Ingredients:

Crust:

1/2 cup slivered almonds

8 teaspoons or 2/3 cup graham cracker crumbs

2 tablespoons sugar

1 tablespoon salted butter, melted

Filling:

1 (8-ounce) packages cream cheese, room temperature

1 (8-ounce) container mascarpone cheese, room temperature

3/4 cup sugar

1 teaspoon fresh lemon juice (I needed to use imitation lemon-juice)

1 teaspoon vanilla extract

2 large eggs, room temperature

Directions

1. Preheat the oven to 350 degrees F. For the crust: You're going to need a 9-inch pan (I had a throw off). Finely grind the almonds, sugar in a food processor, cracker crumbs (I used my Magical Bullet). Add the butter and process until they form moist crumbs.

2. Press the almond mixture on the base of the prepared pan (maybe not on the edges of the pan). Bake the crust until it's set and start to brown, about 1-2 minutes. Cool. Minimize the temperature of the oven to 325 degrees F.

3. For your filling: beat the cream cheese, mascarpone cheese, and sugar in a wide bowl with an electric mixer until smooth, sometimes using a rubber spatula to scrape down the sides of the pot. Beat in the vanilla and lemon juice. Add the eggs, one at a time, beating after each addition until combined.

4. Pour the cheese mixture on the crust from the pan. Put the pan into a large skillet or Pyrex bowl, pour the roasting pan with ample hot water to come halfway up the sides of the skillet. Bake for around 1 hour (the dessert can get tough when it's cold) until the center of the filling shifts slightly when the pan is gently shaken. Move to a stand with the cake; cool for 1 hour. Refrigerate for at least eight hours, until the cheesecake is cold.

5. Topping: squeeze just a small thick cream in the microwave using a chopped Lindt dark chocolate afterward, get a Ziplock baggie and cut out a hole at the corner, then pour the melted chocolate into the baggie and used this to decorate the cake!

Nutrition:

Calories: 148

Sodium: 26 mg

Dietary Fiber: 1.4 g

Total Fat: 3.1 g

Total Carbs: 11.2 g

Protein: 1.6 g

14. Tofu Guacamole

Preparation time: 10 minutes

Cooking time: 30 minutes

Servings: 1

Ingredients:

8oz silken tofu

3 avocados

2 tablespoons fresh coriander (cilantro) chopped

1 bird's-eye chili

Juice of 1 lime

Directions:

1. In a food processor, put all the ingredients and blend a soft chunky consistency with them.

2. Serve with crudités.

Nutrition: Calories: 178

Sodium: 31 mg

Dietary Fiber: 1.2 g

Total Fat: 4.1 g

Total Carbs: 16.6 g

Protein: 1.4 g

15. Chocolate Fondue

Preparation Time: 10 minutes
Cooking Time: 15 minutes
Servings: 1

Ingredients:

4 ounces of dark chocolate min 85% cocoa

11 ounces of strawberries

7 ounces of cherries

2 apples, peeled, cored and sliced

3½ FL oz. double cream, heavy cream

Directions:

1. In a fondue pot or saucepan, place the chocolate and cream then warm it until smooth and creamy.

2. Serve in the fondue pot or transfer it to a serving bowl.

3. Scatter the fruit in a serving dish ready to be dipped into the chocolate.

Nutrition:

Calories: 220,

Sodium: 43 mg,

Dietary Fiber: 5.4 g,

Total Fat: 2.1 g,

Total Carbs: 1.3 g,

Protein: 10.3 g.

16. Choc Nut Truffles

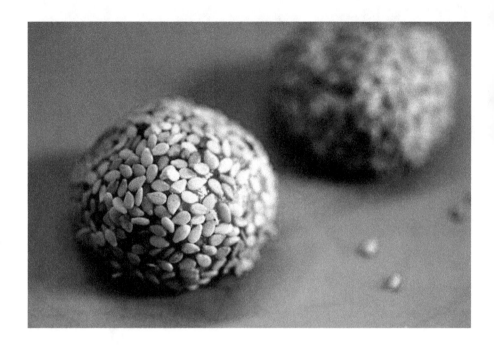

Preparation Time: 10 minutes

Cooking Time: 15 minutes

Servings: 1

Ingredients:

5 ounces of desiccated shredded coconut

2 ounces of walnuts, chopped

1 ounce of hazelnuts, chopped

4 Medjool dates

2 tablespoons 100% cocoa powder or cacao nibs

1 tablespoon coconut oil

Directions:

1. Place ingredients into a blender and process until smooth and creamy.

2. Using a teaspoon, scoop the mixture into bite-size pieces, then roll it into balls.

3. Place them into small paper cases, cover them and chill for 1 hour before serving.

Nutrition:

Calories: 220,

Sodium: 43 mg,

Dietary Fiber: 5.4 g,

Total Fat: 2.1 g,

Total Carbs: 1.3 g,

Protein: 10.3 g.

17. No-Bake Strawberry Flapjacks

Preparation Time: 10 minutes
Cooking Time: 0 minutes
Servings: 1

Ingredients

3 ounces of porridge oats

4 ounces of dates

2 ounces of strawberries

2 ounces of peanuts, unsalted

2 ounces of walnuts

1 tablespoon coconut oil

2 tablespoons 100% cocoa powder or cacao nibs

Directions:

1. Place the ingredients into a blender and process until they become a soft consistency.

2. On a baking sheet or small flat tin, spread the mixture.

3. Press the mixture down and smooth it out.

4. Cut it into 8 pieces, ready to serve.

5. You can add an extra sprinkling of cocoa powder to garnish if you wish.

Nutrition:

Calories: 123

Sodium: 30 mg

Dietary Fiber: 1.4 g

Total Fat: 2.1 g

Total Carbs: 11.3 g

Protein: 1.3 g

18. Dark Chocolate Pretzel Cookies

Preparation time: 10 minutes

Cooking time: 20 minutes

Servings: 2

Ingredients:

1 cup yogurt

1/2 teaspoon baking soda

1/4 teaspoon salt

1/4 teaspoon cinnamon

4 tablespoons butter (softened/0

1/3 cup brown sugar

1 egg

1/2 teaspoon vanilla

1/2 cup dark chocolate chips

1/2 cup pretzels, chopped

Directions

1. Preheat oven to 350 degrees.

2. Whisk the sugar, butter, vanilla and egg together in a medium dish.

3. In another dish, stir the flour, baking soda, and salt together.

4. Stir the bread mixture in, using all the wet components, along with the chocolate chips and pretzels until just blended.

5. Drop large spoonful of dough on an unlined baking sheet.

6. Bake for 15-17 minutes, or until all of the bottoms are crispy.

7. Allow cooling on a wire rack.

Nutrition:
Calories: 150
Sodium: 28 mg
Dietary Fiber: 1.7 g
Total Fat: 4.1 g
Total Carbs: 16.7 g
Protein: 1.4 g

19. Matcha With Vanilla

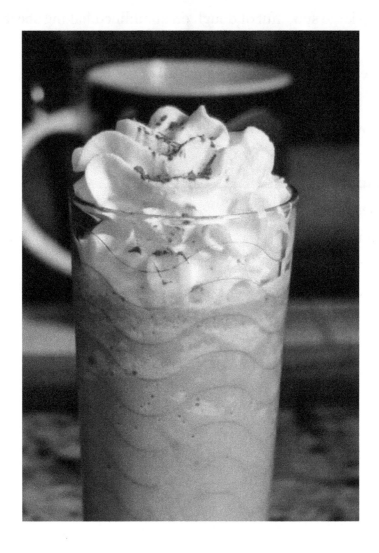

Preparation Time: 5 Minutes,

Cooking time: 0 minutes

Servings: 1

Swap the tasty green matcha and the white tea in this Japanese-style tea or coffee. It's easy to make, and it just takes 5 minutes to make it at home.

Ingredients:

Seeds from half a vanilla pod

½ teaspoon of matcha powder

Directions

1. Heat the kettle, then apply 100ml of water to it. In a tiny cup, pour half the hot water, steam and then transfer the matcha powder and vanilla seeds to the remaining water in the cup.

2. Stir the mixture up to a smooth, slightly smooth and lump-free matcha with a bamboo whisk or mini-electric whisk. In the hot teapot, remove the water and then dump the cooked matcha tea into it. Prefer, with sweet honey or agave.

Nutrition:

Calories: 210

Sodium: 34 mg

Dietary Fiber: 1.4 g

Total Fat: 4.3 g

Total Carbs: 15.3 g

Protein: 1.6 g

20. Warm Berries & Cream

Preparation Time: 10 minutes

Cooking Time: 15 minutes

Servings: 1

Ingredients:

9 ounces of blueberries

9 ounces of strawberries

3 ounces of. Red currants

3ounce of blackberries

Tablespoons fresh whipped cream

1 tablespoon honey

Directions:

1. Mix all ingredients into a bowl.

2. Scoop out a little of the mixture and shape it into a ball.

3. Roll the ball in a little cocoa powder and set aside.

4. Repeat for the remaining mixture. It can be consumed immediately or kept in the fridge.

Nutrition:

Calories: 193

Sodium: 32 mg

Dietary Fiber: 1.4 g

Total Fat: 4.6 g

Total Carbs: 16.8 g

Protein: 1.6 g

21. Home-Made Ice-Cream Drumsticks

Preparation time: 30 minutes

Cooking time: 0 minute

Servings: 2

Ingredients:

Vanilla ice cream

Two Lindt hazelnut chunks

Magical shell - out chocolate

Sugar levels

Nuts (I mixed crushed peppers and unsalted peanuts)

Parchment paper

Directions:

1. Soften ice cream and mixing topping and two sliced of hazelnut balls.

2. Fill underside of Magic shell with sugar and nuts and top with ice-cream.

3. Wrap parchment paper round cone and then fill cone over about 1.5 inches across the cap of the cone (the paper can help to carry its shape).

4. Sprinkle with magical nuts and shells.

5. Freeze for about 20 minutes, before the ice cream is eaten.

Nutrition:

Calories: 153

Sodium: 32 mg

Dietary Fiber: 1.4 g

Total Fat: 4.1 g

Total Carbs: 16.3 g

Protein: 1.6 g

22. Mocha Chocolate Mousse

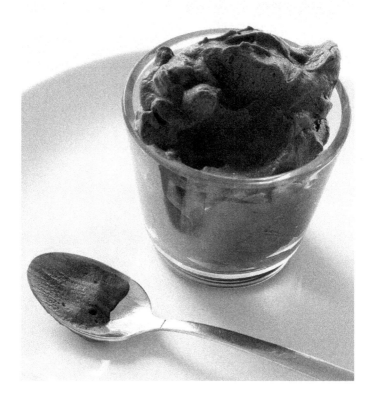

Preparation time: 15 minutes

Cooking time: 2 hours

Dish out s 4-- 6.

Ingredients:

250g dark chocolate (85% cocoa solids)

6 medium free-range eggs, separated

4 table spoon strong black coffee

4 table spoon almond milk

Chocolate coffee beans, to embellish

Directions:

Melt the chocolate in a big bowl set over a pan of gently simmering water, ensuring the bottom of the bowl does not touch the water. Eliminate the bowl from the first heat and leave the melted chocolate to cool to space temperature level.

When the melted chocolate is at space temperature, whisk in the egg yolks one at a time and then carefully fold in the coffee and almond milk.

Using a hand-held electric mixer, blend the egg whites up until stiff peaks form, then blend a couple of tablespoons into the chocolate mixture to loosen it. Carefully fold in the rest, using a big metal spoon.

Transfer the mousse to individual glasses and smooth the surface area. Cover with stick film and chill for a minimum of 2 hours, ideally overnight. Decorate with chocolate coffee beans prior to serving.

23. Best Banana Bread Ever

Preparation time: 15 minutes

Cooking time: 45 minutes

Ingredients:

150 g unsalted butter melted

200 g self-raising flour I utilized brown 1/2 teaspoon bicarbonate of soda 1/2 teaspoon salt

150 g light soft brown sugar or caster sugar

2 large eggs

4 ripe bananas mashed

50 g combined seeds or nuts optional

Directions:

Prefirst heat your microwave oven to 320F.

Place the butter in a little saucepan and melt carefully on a low very first heat. When all the butter is melted. Turn off and leave to cool for a few minutes.

Line 2 little (1lb) loaf tins with greaseproof paper. Scrunch up a sheet of greaseproof paper big enough to fit in one of your loaf tins. Wet it under the cold tap then utilize it to line the loaf tin. Repeat with the other tin.

Next, tip the flour into a big bowl and include the bicarbonate of salt, soda and sugar. Stir to integrate.

Peel the bananas and rip them into pieces. Location the banana chunks in a small bowl or container. Utilize a potato masher to mash them approximately then include the eggs and stir to combine.

Idea the eggs and banana mix into the dry things r eq uired and stir completely up until you have a thick batter. Consist of the cooled melted butter and stir well.

Consist of the nuts or seeds, if you are utilizing them, and stir as soon as more till the seeds are uniformly dispersed.

Divide the mix between the 2 loaf tins and cook the banana bread in your prefirst heated microwave oven for 45 minutes. If not prepare your banana bread for a more 5 minutes and examine again.

When your banana bread is prepared. Eliminate from the microwave oven. Allow to cool for 5 minutes then remove from the tin, peel off the greaseproof paper and cool on a cake rack ... or enjoy while it is still warm!

24. Raw Brownie Bites

Preparation time: 2,50 hours

Ingredients:

Whole walnuts 2½ cups

Almonds ¼ cup

Medjool dates 2½ cups

Cacao powder 1 cup

Vanilla extract one teaspoon

Sea salt ⅛-¼ teaspoon

Directions:

Place all once well mixed in a food processor.

Place on a baking sheet and freeze for 30 minutes, or 2 hours in the refrigerator. Roll yourself into balls.

25. Avocado Mayo Medley

Preparation time: 5 minutes

Cooking time: 0 minutes

Servings: 3

Ingredients:

1 medium avocado, cut into chunks

½ teaspoon ground cayenne pepper

2 tablespoons fresh cilantro ¼ cup olive oil

½ cup mayo, low fat and los sodium

Directions:

Take a food processor and add avocado, cayenne pepper, lime juice, salt and cilantro.

Mix until smooth.

Slowly incorporate olive oil add 1 tablespoon at a time and keep processing between additions. Store and use as needed!

26. Hearty Almond Crackers

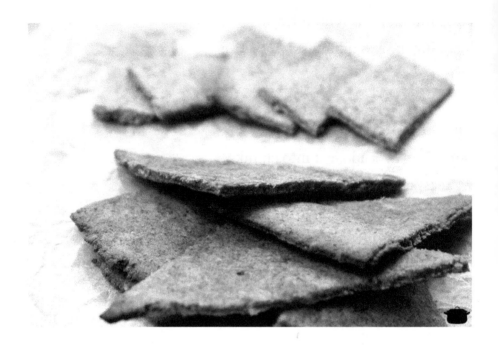

Preparation time: 10 minutes

Cooking Time: 20 minutes

Ingredients:

1 cup almond flour

1⁄4 teaspoon of baking soda and 1/8 teaspoon of black pepper

3 tablespoons sesame seeds

1 egg, beaten

Salt and pepper to taste

Directions:

Preheat to 350 degrees F in your oven.

Line two parchment paper baking sheets and hold them on one side.

Break the dough into 2 balls.

Roll the dough in between two parchment paper bits.

Break the crackers and pass them on to the baking sheet that has been prepared.

For 15-20 minutes, bake.

Repeat until all of the dough has been used up.

Leave crackers to cool and serve.

Enjoy!

27. Black Bean Salsa

Preparation time: 5 minutes

Cooking time: 0 minutes

Servings: 3

Ingredients:

1 tablespoon coconut aminos

½ teaspoon cumin, ground

1 cup canned black beans, no salt

1 cup of salsa

6 cups romaine lettuce, torn

½ cup avocado, peeled, pitted and cubed

Directions:

Take a bowl and add beans, alongside other ingredients.

Toss well and serve.

Enjoy!

28. Corn Spread

Preparation time: 5 minutes

Cooking time: 0 minutes

Servings: 3

Ingredients:

30 ounce canned corn, drained

2 green onions, chopped

½ cup coconut cream

1 jalapeno, chopped

½ teaspoon chili powder

Directions:

Take a pan and add corn, green onions, jalapeno, chili powder, stir well.

Bring to a simmer over medium heat and cook for 10 minutes.

Let it chill and add coconut cream.

Stir well.

Serve and enjoy!

29. Special Green Tea Smoothie

Preparation time: 10 Minutes

Cooking Time: 0 Minutes

Servings 2

Ingredients:

250 ml milk

2 ripe bananas

1/2 tsp vanilla bean paste

2 teaspoons of honey

6 ice cubes

2 teaspoons of matcha green tea powder

Directions:

Using a blender or smoothie machine, combine all the ingredients together. Enjoy and serve.

30. Special Blackcurrant and Oat Yoghurt

Preparation time: 10 Minutes

Cooking Time: 0 Minutes

Servings 4

Ingredients:

400 grams of greek yogurt, plain

200g blackcurrants, washed and stalks removed

200 ml of water

4 tablespoon of caster sugar (or your own choice of sweetener)

80 grams of oats

Directions:

In a small pan, simply place the blackcurrants, water, and sugar. Bring to boil.

After boiling, slightly reduce the heat, maintain the simmer and cook for another 4 to 5 minutes.

Turn off the heat and allow it to cool the mixture.

After cooling, you can now refrigerate your blackcurrant compote until ready to be used.

Using a large bowl, place the yogurt and oats, then thoroughly stir in together.

Divide the blackcurrant compote into 4 serving bowls, then just a simple top with the oats and yogurt. Mix and enjoy.

31. Fruit & Nut Yoghurt Crunch

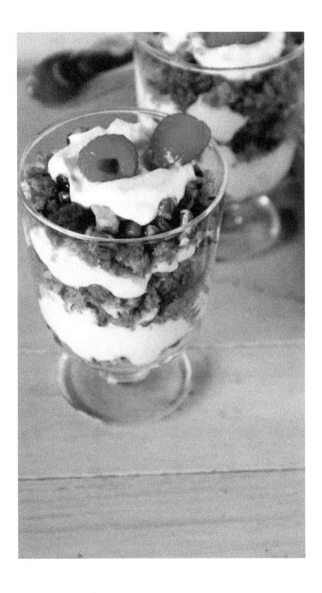

Preparation time: 5 minutes

Cooking time: 25 minutes

Servings: 4

Ingredients:

100g (3½ oz) plain Greek yogurt

50g (2oz) strawberries, chopped

6 walnut halves, chopped

Sprinkling of cocoa powder

Directions:

1. Stir half of the chopped strawberries into the yogurt.

2. Using a glass, place a layer of yogurt with a sprinkling of strawberries and walnuts, followed by another layer of the same until you reach the top of the glass.

3. Garnish with walnuts pieces and a dusting of cocoa powder.

32. Fruity Granola Bars

Preparation time: 5 minutes

Cooking time: 30 minutes

Servings: 3

Ingredients:

¾ cup packed brown sugar ½ cup honey

¼ cup water

1 teaspoon salt

½ cup cocoa butter 3 cups rolled oats

1 cup walnuts, chopped

1 cup ground buckwheat ¼ cup sesame seeds

½ cup dried strawberries or mixed fruits ½ cup raisins

½ cup Medjool dates, chopped

Directions:

In a large pan, combine sugar, cocoa butter, honey, water, and salt. Bring to a simmer and cook for 5 minutes.

Score deeply into bars roughly 2" wide by 4" tall.

Allow cooling for 30 minutes before breaking or cutting along score lines. Store in an airtight container.

33. Cardamom Granola Bars

Preparation time: 5 minutes

Cooking time: 30 minutes

Servings: 3

Ingredients:

2 cups rolled oats

½ cup raisins

½ cup walnuts, chopped and toasted

1 ½ teaspoon ground cardamom

6 tablespoons cocoa butter 1/3 cup packed brown sugar 3 tablespoons honey Coconut oil, for greasing pan

Directions:

Preheat the oven to 350°F.

With foil, line a 9-inch square pan, spreading the foil over the edges. Grease the coconut oil on the foil.

Mix the oats, raisins, walnuts and cardamom in a large bowl.

Heat the cocoa butter, brown sugar and honey in a saucepan until the butter melts and begins to bubble.

Bake on top for approximately 30 minutes or until golden brown. Enable it to cool for 30 minutes. With the foil, lift the granola out of the pan, place the cutting board on and put it on. Cut into 18 bars.

34. Coconut Brownie Bites

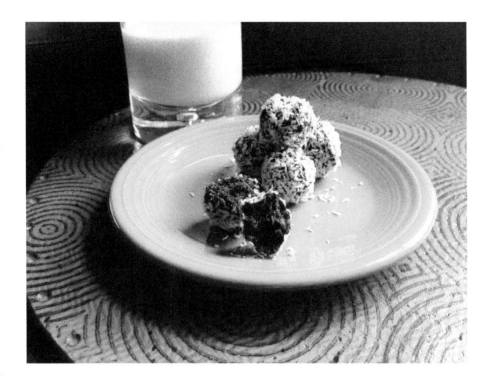

Preparation time: 5 minutes

Cooking time: 40 minutes

Servings: 3

Ingredients:

¼ cup unsweetened cocoa powder

¼ cup unsweetened desiccated or shredded coconut

Directions:

In a food processor, put everything and blend until well combined.

Roll into 1" balls.

Roll balls in coconut until well-covered and place on a wax paper-lined baking sheet.

Freeze for 30 minutes or refrigerate for up to 2 hours.

35. Tortilla Chips and Fresh Salsa

Preparation time: 5 minutes

Cooking time: 50 minutes

Servings: 3

Ingredients:

4 whole wheat flour tortillas

2 tablespoons extra virgin olive oil

4 Roma tomatoes, diced

1 small red onion, finely diced

1 Bird's Eye chili pepper, finely diced

2 teaspoons parsley, finely chopped

2 teaspoons cilantro, finely chopped

1 lime, juiced

Salt and pepper to taste

Directions:

Preheat oven to 350 degrees F.

Cover one side of each tortilla in olive oil using a pastry brush.

Divide each tortilla into 8 wedges with a sharp knife or pizza cutter. Spread the tortillas in a single layer over a large baking sheet. If possible, use more than one baking sheet. Bake for 8 to 10 minutes, until both sides are golden brown and your chips are crispy, flipping halfway through.

While the chips are baking, combine tomatoes, red onion, chili pepper, parsley, cilantro and lime juice and mix well.

Serve salsa with the chips.

36. The Bell Pepper Fiesta

Preparation time: 5 minutes

Cooking time: 0 minutes

Servings: 3

Ingredients:

2 tablespoons dill, chopped

1 yellow onion, chopped

1 pound multicolored peppers, cut, halved, seeded and cut into thin strips

3 tablespoons organic olive oil

2 ½ tablespoons white wine vinegar

Black pepper to taste

Directions:

Take a bowl and mix in sweet pepper, onion, dill, pepper, oil, vinegar and toss well.

Divide between bowls and serve.

Enjoy!

37. Spiced Up Pumpkin Seeds Bowls

Preparation time: 5 minutes

Cooking time: 30 minutes

Servings: 3

Ingredients:

½ tablespoon chili powder

½ teaspoon cayenne

2 cups pumpkin seeds

2 teaspoons lime juice

Directions:

Spread pumpkin seeds over a lined baking sheet, add lime juice, cayenne and chili powder.Toss well.

Preheat your oven to 275 degrees F.

Roast in your oven for 20 minutes and transfer to small bowls.

Serve and enjoy!

38. Mozzarella Cauliflower Bars

Preparation time: 5 minutes

Cooking time: 30 minutes

Servings: 3

Ingredients:

1 cauliflower head, riced

12 cup low-fat mozzarella cheese, shredded ¼ cup egg whites

1 teaspoon Italian dressing, low fat

Pepper to taste

Directions:

Spread over a lined baking sheet with cauliflower rice.

Preheat your oven to 375 degrees F.

Roast for 20 minutes.

Transfer to bowl and spread pepper, cheese, seasoning, egg whites and stir well.

Spread in a rectangular pan and press.

Transfer to the oven and cook for an additional 20 minutes.

Serve and enjoy!

39. Feta and Beet Stacked Appetizer

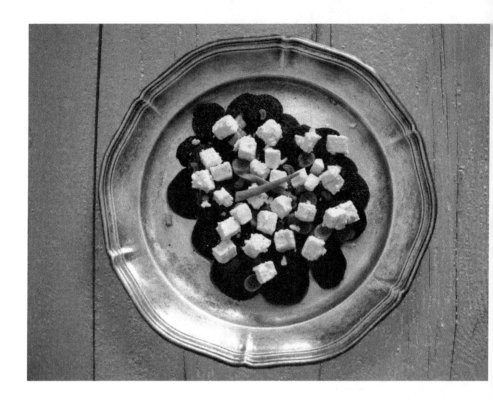

Preparation time: 5 minutes

Cooking time: 20 minutes

Servings: 4

Ingredients:

2 large fresh beets

½ teaspoon dried lovage

½ cup red wine vinegar

¼ cup lemon juice (optional) ½ cup feta cheese

½ cup walnuts, crushed

Directions:

Soak the lovage in the red wine vinegar while you're preparing the rest of the appetizer.

Bring a pot of water to a boil and cook the beets for 25 minutes or until they are tender.

Cool, peel, and slice in 1/3" thick slices.

Place beets in a bowl with the lovage red wine vinegar and marinate 15 minutes.

Separate the beets from the vinegar and add the lemon juice to the liquid. Place a few beet slices on a microwave-safe dish and sprinkle them with some feta cheese and crushed walnuts. Drizzle with some of the lemon vinegar mixes.

Top with more beet slices, and sprinkle again with feta, walnuts and lemon vinegar. Repeat until you have no more beet slices left.

Microwave for 45 seconds to 1 minute on medium.

Cool slightly before serving.

40. Blueberry Nut Bran Muffins

Preparation time: 5 minutes

Cooking time: 10 minutes

Servings: 4

Ingredients:

Wheat bran – 1 cup

Whole wheat flour – 1.5 cups

Sea salt - .5 teaspoon

Baking soda - .25 teaspoon

Baking powder - .25 teaspoon

Cinnamon – 1.5 teaspoons

Eggs – 2

Soy milk, unsweetened - .75 cup

Apple cider vinegar – 1 tablespoon

Apple sauce, unsweetened - .33 cup

Date sugar – .5 cup

Soybean oil - .33 cup

Blueberries, fresh or frozen – 1 cup

Walnuts, chopped - .5 cup

Directions:

Begin by setting your standard or toaster oven to Fahrenheit four-hundred degrees. Line a twelve-cup muffin tin and then spray the paper liners with nonstick cooking spray.

Whisk together the eggs, applesauce, date sugar, soybean oil, soy milk, and apple cider vinegar in a large bowl until fully combined. Set it aside.

In another clean cup, whisk together the whole wheat flour, wheat bran, cinnamon, sea salt, baking soda, and baking soda. Once the dry ingredients are combined, fol them into the other prepared ingredients. Gently fold in the blueberries and walnuts, just until combined.

Divide the blueberry nut bran muffin batter between the prepared muffin liners and allow them to cook until fully done and a toothpick once inserted is removed clean, about fifteen to eighteen minutes. Enable the muffins to cool for five minutes before removing them from the oven.

Withdrawing them from the pan.

41. Plum Oat Bars

Preparation time: 5 minutes

Cooking time: 10 minutes

Servings: 4

Ingredients:

Rolled oats – 1.5 cups

Baking powder – 1 teaspoon

Almond meal - .5 cup

Cinnamon – 1.5 teaspoon

Soybean oil – 2 tablespoons

Sea salt - .25 teaspoon

Prunes – 2 cups

Directions:

Begin by preheating the oven to Fahrenheit three-hundred and fifty degrees and preparing the prunes. Add the prunes to a large bowl and pour hot water over them until fully submerged.

Allow the prunes to sit in the water for five minutes, until soft.

Remove the prunes from the water and transfer them to a blender or food processor, reserving the water. Pour in a small amount of the water that you previously reserved from the prunes and blend until the prunes form a thick paste.

Add two tablespoons of the prepared prune puree to a medium kitchen bowl along with the oil, sea salt, baking powder, cinnamon, almond flour, and rolled oats. Combine together until the mixture resembles a crumble, slightly like wet sand. You can add more prune puree if it is too dry.

Line a square baking dish with kitchen parchment and then press three-quarters of the oat mixture into the bottom to form a crust. Spread the remaining prune puree over the top of the crust, and then sprinkle the remaining oat mixture over the prune puree to add a crumble.

Cook the bars in the oven until set and slightly toasted, about fifteen minutes. Remove the plum oat bars from the hot oven and let the pan cool completely. After the bars have reached room temperature slice them into nine bars and enjoy.

42. Spinach and Kale Mix

Preparation time: 5 minutes

Cooking time: 30 minutes

Servings: 4

Ingredients:

2 chopped shallots

1 c. no-salt-added and chopped canned tomatoes

2 c. baby spinach

2 minced garlic cloves

5 c. torn kale

1 tbsp. olive oil

Directions:

Heat up a pan with the oil over medium-high heat, add the shallots, stir and sauté for 5 minutes.

Add the spinach, kale and the other ingredients, toss, cook for 10 minutes more, divide between plates and serve.

43. Kale Dip with Cajun Pita Chips

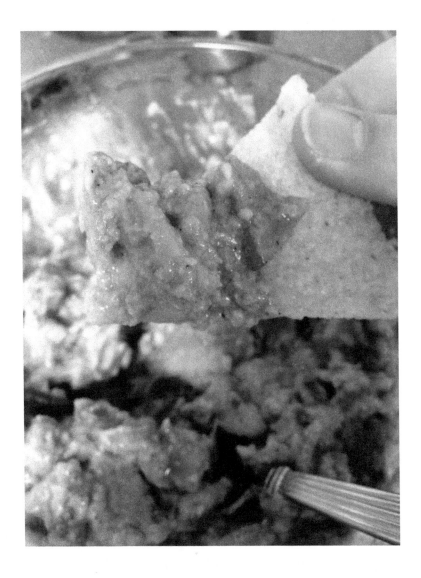

Preparation time: 10 minutes

Baking time: 8 – 10 minutes

Cooking time: 1 hour

Ingredients:

For the Dip:

2 cups sour cream

1 ½ cups baby kale

¼ cup red bell pepper, diced

¼ cup green onions, diced

1 clove garlic, minced

1/8 teaspoon chili pepper flakes

For the Chips:

5 pita bread, halved and split open

½ cup extra virgin olive oil

½ teaspoon Cajun seasoning ¼ teaspoon ground cumin ¼ teaspoon turmeric

Salt to taste

Directions:

To make the dip: In a bowl, combine the sour cream, baby kale, red pepper, onions, garlic, salt and chili pepper flakes. Cover and refrigerate for at least 1 hour. For the processing of chips: Preheat the oven to 400 degrees F.

Break half of each pita into four wedges. Combine the Cajun seasoning, olive oil, cumin and turmeric and brush over the rough side of the wedges of the pita. Place on ungreased baking sheets and cook for 8-10 minutes or until golden brown and crisp chips are available. Serve with dip.

44. Snack Bites

Preparation Time: 5 Minutes

Cooking time: 35 Minutes

Servings: 2

Ingredients:

120g walnuts

30g dark chocolate (85% cocoa)

250g dates

1 tablespoon pure cocoa powder

1 tablespoon turmeric

1 tablespoon of olive oil

Directions:

Contents of a pod of vanilla or other flavoring of vanilla

Coarsely crumble the chocolate and mix it with the walnuts in a food processor into a fine powder.

Then add the other ingredients and stir until you have a uniform dough. If necessary, add 1 to 2 tablespoons of water.

Form 15 pieces from the mixture and refrigerate in an airtight tin for at least one hour.

The bites will remain in the refrigerator for a week.

45. Spinach Mix

Preparation time: 10 minutes
Cooking time: 12 minutes
Servings: 4

Ingredients:

1 pound baby spinach
1 yellow onion, chopped
1 tablespoon olive oil
1 tablespoon lemon juice
2 garlic cloves, minced
A pinch of cayenne pepper
¼ teaspoon smoked paprika

Directions:

Heat up a pan with the oil over medium-high heat, add the onion and the
garlic and sauté for 2 minutes.
Add the cooked spinach for 10 minutes over medium heat, divide between
Plates and as a side dish to eat.

46. Walnut Stuffed Bacon Wrapped Dates

Preparation time: 10 - 20minutes

Baking time: 10 minutes

Servings: 4

Ingredients:

4 ounces walnuts, halved

Directions:

Preheat your broiler.

Slit the dates and place one walnut half inside each. Wrap dates with ½ slice of bacon, using

toothpicks to hold them together.

Broil 10 minutes, turning once, or until bacon is evenly brown and crisp.

47. Loaded Chocolate Fudge

Preparation time: 10 minutes

Cooking Time: 1+ hours

Ingredients:

1 cup Medjool dates, chopped

2 tablespoons coconut oil, melted

1/2 cup peanut butter

¼ cup of unsweetened cocoa powder ½ cup walnuts

1 teaspoon vanilla

Directions:

Lightly grease an 8' square baking pan with coconut oil and soak the dates in warm water for 20-30 minutes.

Add dates, peanut butter, cocoa powder and vanilla to a food processer and blend until smooth. Fold in walnuts.

Pack into the greased baking pan and put in your freezer for 1 hour or until fudge is solid and firm.

Cut into 16 or more bite-sized squares and store in semi-airtight container in the refrigerator.

48. Kale Chips

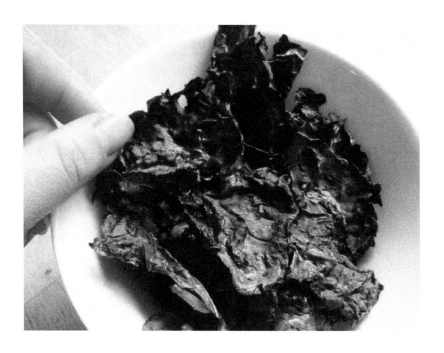

Preparation Time: 5 Minutes

Cooking time: 55 Minutes

Servings: 2

Ingredients:

1 large head of curly kale, wash, dry and pulled from stem 1 tbsp.
extra virgin

olive oil

Minced parsley

A squeeze of lemon juice

Cayenne pepper (just a pinch)

Dash of soy sauce

Directions:

In a large bowl, rip the kale from the stem into palm-sized pieces. Sprinkle the minced parsley, olive oil, soy sauce, a squeeze of the lemon juice, and a very small pinch of the cayenne powder.

Toss with a set of tongs or salad forks, and make sure to coat all of the leaves.

If you have a dehydrator, turn it on to 118 F, spread out the kale on a dehydrator sheet, and leave in there for about 2 hours.

If you are cooking them, place parchment paper on top of a cookie sheet. Lay the bed of kale and separate it a bit to make sure the kale is evenly toasted. Cook for 10-15 minutes maximum at 250F.

49. Moroccan Leeks Snack

Preparation time: 5 minutes

Cooking time: 0 minutes

Servings: 3

Ingredients:

1 bunch radish, sliced

3 cups leeks, chopped

1 ½ cups olives, pitted and sliced

Pinch turmeric powder

2 tablespoons essential olive oil

1 cup cilantro, chopped

Directions:

Take a bowl and mix in radishes, leeks, olives and cilantro.

Mix well.

Season with pepper, oil, turmeric and toss well.

Serve and enjoy!

50. Honey Nuts

Preparation Time: 5 Minutes

Cooking time: 35 Minutes

Servings: 2

Ingredients:

150g (5oz) walnuts

150g (5oz) pecan nuts

50g (2oz) softened butter

1 tablespoon honey

½ bird's-eye chili, very finely chopped and deseeded

Directions:

Preheat the 180C/360F oven. In a cup, mix the butter, honey and chili and add the nuts and stir well. Spread the nuts over a lined baking sheet and roast for 10 minutes in the oven, stirring halfway through once. Take it out of the oven and allow it to cool before eating.

CPSIA information can be obtained
at www.ICGtesting.com
Printed in the USA
BVHW011015150321
602551BV00001B/56

9 781801 452908